Emily Gilmore

INTERMITTENT FASTING FOR WOMEN OVER 50: THE PERFECT SOLUTION

The complete and easy guide to Fight Aging, get Healty, Strong and Slim Again Without feeling Hungry.

Table of Contents

Introduction

Intermittent fasting (IF) is just a method for partitioning your meal plans into times of eating and fasting.

Intermittent fasting for women over 50 has been clinically demonstrated to upgrade the skeletal framework's overall well-being. It has been seen as a productive method for diminishing the indications of joint inflammation and back agony, which more seasoned women usually experience. A couple of studies have additionally demonstrated how changing meal plans as per IF can influence the generation of hormones that control muscle and bone wellbeing.

For women over 50, this method can also help expand confidence and better mind-sets alongside a reduction in negative manifestations like uneasiness, despair, and stress.

2

Eating during specific timeframes is associated with a diminished danger of diabetes. A few investigations show that intermittent fasting can be a productive method to hold glucose levels under tight restraints, get off insulin, and even dispose of or decrease the use of recommending medications.

When a woman begins fasting at fixed interims, her body begins sending a sign that actuates a hereditary fix instrument. This system battles maturing and different sicknesses by delivering human development hormone (HGH). Thus, HGH attempts to strengthen muscles, tendons, and ligaments, accelerate metabolic rate, recover tissues, and increment life span. This is ostensibly probably the best bit of leeway of intermittent fasting for women over 50.

Being perhaps the most sizzling theme in the weight loss world, intermittent fasting has substantiated itself as a fruitful solution for getting thinner, keeping up bulk, expanding life span, and in any

3

event, upgrading discernment. Most importantly, it is considered broadly valuable for more established women who need to lose paunch fat.

Chapter 1: What is Intermittent Fasting and its Types

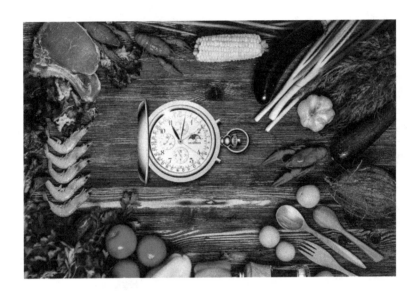

Intermittent fasting is an eating pattern where a person cycles between eating and fasting periods. Therefore, it is more of a way of eating than a diet.

Intermittent fasting is not as hard as you may think. If anything, it is the exact opposite. There is less planning involved, and many people who have practiced it say that they feel more energetic and generally good during the fast. It may be challenging when starting, but the body quickly adapts, and you get used to it.

Types of Intermittent Fasting

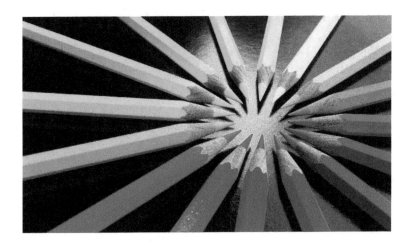

16/8 Method

This's just about the most popular fasting methods since it's so schedule-based, meaning there are no surprises. This will give you the freedom to control when you eat based on the everyday life of yours. The sixteen is the number of hours you're likely to be fasting, which may also be lowered to twelve or perhaps fourteen hours if that fits into your life better. Then your eating period is going to be between eight and ten hours every day. This might seem daunting, but it just means that you are skipping an entire meal. Many people choose to begin their fast around 7 or 8 p.m. and then do not eat until 11 or noon the next day, which means they fast for the recommended 16 hours. Of course, it isn't as bad as it sounds since they are sleeping during this time, so what it comes down to is eating dinner and then not eating again the next day around lunch, so you are just skipping breakfast.

You will be doing it every day, so finding the hours that work for you are important. If you work the third shift, then switching your eating period to fit into your schedule is important. If you find yourself running down and sluggish, tweak your fasting hours until you find a healthy balance. Granted, there will be some adjustment, because, chances are, your body is not accustomed to skipping entire meals. However, this should go away after a couple of weeks. If it doesn't then try starting your fasting period earlier in the day, allowing you to eat earlier or alter it, you need to feel healthy and happy.

Lean-Gains Method (14:10)

The lean-gains method has several different incarnations on the web, but its fame comes from the fact that it helps shed fat while building it into muscle almost immediately. Through the lean-gains method, you'll find yourself able to shift all that fat to be muscle through a rigorous practice of fasting, eating right, and exercising.

Through this method, you fast anywhere from 14 to 16 hours and spend the remaining 10 or 8 hours each day engaged in eating and exercise. As opposed to the crescendo, this method features daily fasting and eating, rather than alternated eating days versus not. Therefore, you don't have to be quite cautious about extending the physical effort to exercise on the days you are fasting because those days when you're fasting are every day!

For the lean-gaining method, start fasting only for 14 hours and work it up to 16 if you feel comfortable with it, but never forget to drink enough water and be careful about spending too much energy on exercise! Remember that you want to grow in health and potential through intermittent fasting. You'll certainly not want to lose any of that growth by forcing the process along.

20:4 Method

Stepping things up a notch from the 14:10 and 16:8 methods, the 20:4 method is a tough one to master, for it is rather unforgiving. People talk about this method of intermittent fasting as intense and highly restrictive. Still, they also say that the effects of living this method are almost unparalleled with all other tactics.

For the 20:4 method, you'll fast for 20 hours each day and squeeze all your meals, all your eating, and all your snacking into 4 hours. People who attempt 20:4 normally have two smaller meals or just one large meal and a few snacks during their 4-hour window to eat, and it is up to the individual which four hours of the day they devote to eating.

The trick for this method is to make sure you're not overeating or bingeing during those 4-hour windows to eat. It is all-too-easy to get hungry during the 20-hour fast and have that feeling then propel you into intense and unrealistic hunger or meal sizes after the fast period is over. Be careful if you try this method. If you're new to intermittent fasting, work your way up to this one gradually, and if you're working your way up already, only make the shift to 20:4 when you know you're ready. It would surely disappoint if all your progress with intermittent fasting got hijacked by one poorly thought-out goal with 20:4 method.

Meal Skipping

Meal skipping is an extremely flexible form of intermittent fasting that can provide all of the benefits of intermittent fasting but with a less strict schedule. If you are not someone who has a typical schedule or feels like a more strict variation of the intermittent fasting diet will serve you, meal skipping is a viable alternative.

Many people who choose to use meal skipping find it a great way to listen to their bodies and follow their basic instincts. If they are not hungry, they simply don't eat that meal. Instead, they wait for the next one. Meal skipping can also help people who have time constraints and who may not always get in a certain meal of the day.

It is important to realize that you may not always be maintaining a 10–16-hour window of fasting with meal skipping. As a result, you may not get every benefit that comes from other fasting diets. However, this may be a great solution for people

12

who want an intermittent fasting diet that feels more natural. It may also be a great idea for those looking to begin listening to their bodies more so that they can adjust to a more intense variation of the diet with greater ease. It can be a great transitional diet for you if you are not ready to jump into one of the other fasting diets just yet.

Warrior Diet Fasting

The most extreme form of intermittent fasting is known as the Warrior Diet. This intermittent fasting cycle follows a 20-hour fasting window with a short 4-hour eating window. During that eating window, individuals are supposed only to consume raw fruits and vegetables. They can also eat one large meal. Typically, the eating window occurs at nighttime so people can snack throughout the evening, have a large meal, and then resume fasting.

Because of the fasting length of the Warrior Diet, people should also consume a fairly hearty level of healthy fats. Doing so will give the body something to consume during the fast to produce energy with. A small number of carbohydrates can also be incorporated to support energy levels, too.

People who eat the Warrior Diet tend to believe that humans are natural nocturnal eaters and are not meant to eat throughout the day. The belief is that eating this way follows our natural circadian rhythms, allowing our body to work optimally.

The only people who should consider doing the Warrior Diet have already had success with other forms of intermittent fasting and who are used to it. Attempting to jump straight into the Warrior Diet can have serious repercussions for anyone who is not used to intermittent fasting. Even still, those used to it may find this particular style too extreme for them to maintain.

Eat-Stop-Eat (24 Hour) Method

This method of fasting is incredibly similar to the crescendo method. The only discernable difference is that there's no anticipation of increasing into a more intense fasting pattern with time. For the eat-stop-eat method, you decide which days you want to take off from eating, and then you run with it until you've lost that weight and then keep running with the lifestyle for good because you won't be able to imagine life without it.

The eat-stop-eat method involves one to two days a week being 100% oriented towards fasting, with the other five to six days concerning "business as normal." The one or two days spent fasting are then full 24-hour days spent without eating anything at all. These days, of course, water and coffee are still fine to drink, but no food items can be consumed whatsoever. Exercise is also frowned upon on those fasting days but see what your body can handle before deciding how that should all work out.

15

Some people might start thinking they're using the crescendo method but end up sticking with eat-stop-eat.

Alternate-Day Method

The alternate-day method is admittedly a little confusing, but the reason it could be so confusing could come, in part, from how much wiggle room it provides for the practitioner. This method is great for people who don't have a consistent schedule or any sense of one, it is incredibly forgiving for those who don't quite have everything together for themselves yet.

When it comes down to it, alternate-day intermittent fasting is really up to you. You should try to fast every other day, but it doesn't have to be that precise. Similarly, with the crescendo method, as long as you fast two to three days a week, with a break day or two in between each fasting day, you're set! Then, you'll want to eat normally for three or four days out of each week, and when you encounter a fasting day, you don't even need to completely fast!

Alternate-day fasting is a solid place to start from, especially if you work a varying schedule or still have to get used to a consistent one. If you want to make things more intense from this starting point, the alternate-day method can easily become the eat-stop-eat method, the crescendo method, or the 5:2 method. Essentially, this method is a great place to begin

12:12 Method

As another of the more natural ways of intermittent fasting, 12:12 approach is well-suited to beginning practitioners. Many people live out 12:12 method without any forethought simply because of their sleeping and eating schedule but turning 12:12 into a conscious practice can have just as many positive effects on your life as the more drastic 20:4 method claims.

According to a study conducted in the University of Alabama For this method, you fast for 12 hours and then enter a 12-hour eating window. It's not difficult to get three small meals and several snacks, or two big meals and a snack into your day with this method. With the 12:12 method, the standard meal schedule works well.

Ultimately, this method is a great one to start from, for a lot of variation can be built into this scheduling when you're ready to make things more interesting. Effortlessly and without much effort, 12:12 can become 14:10 or even 16:8, and in seemingly no time, you can find yourself trying alternate-day or crescendo methods, too. Start with what's normal for you, and this method might be exactly that!

Chapter 2: Why IF Is Good for Women Over 50

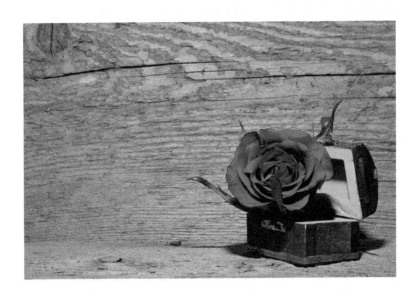

Boost Weight Loss

Most people discover intermittent fasting either because they want to lose weight or gain health benefits. But, sometimes losing weight can accomplish both of those simultaneously, as a high body fat percentage can increase high blood pressure, cholesterol, and early mortality. Whether you are hoping to gain these health benefits by losing weight or wish to lose weight to feel more comfortable in your skin, you will love how intermittent fasting can boost your weight loss.

Balance Important Hormones

Thankfully, studies have found intermittent fasting can help balance a person's cortisol and melioration levels. It does this in a variety of ways. For instance, it can help to reduce cortisol by balancing and regulating blood sugar levels. Balancing cortisol sets off a chain reaction that improves the balance of other hormones, including melatonin. One simple change can benefit many hormones and systems within your body.

Improve Heart Health

As we age, we all must take even more care of our heart health. After all, heart disease is the number one killer of both men and women. While doctors often educate men on the symptoms and warning signs of heart attacks, women are often forgotten, leading to an increased risk of death. This means women must be extra vigilant, taking care of their heart health and educating themselves on the warning signs of heart attacks.

One crucial way to increase heart health is to watch your cholesterol. There is not a single type of cholesterol, but several. The two main types include LDL, known as the "bad" cholesterol, and HDL, known as the "good" cholesterol. While LDL cholesterol will increase your heart attack and heart disease risk, HDL cholesterol will protect your heart and remove LDL cholesterol from your body.

Increase Mental Energy and Efficiency

We all need mental energy to get through the day. When our mind is sluggish, we cannot think, accomplish anything, and sometimes we may be unable even to stay awake. We have all had trouble focusing on work, completing a math problem, remembering what we have read, and so on. This is all due to a lack of mental energy and efficiency. You may think that intermittent fasting would further reduce your mental state, as hunger makes focusing difficult, but the opposite is exact.

Reduce the Potential Risk of Developing Cancer

Of course, nobody can promise that any lifestyle choice will prevent you from developing cancer. However, studies have found that intermittent fasting can potentially reduce your risk. Further studies are ongoing, but current research through animal studies have proven promising. For instance, it was found that rats with tumors survive longer when placed on fasting schedules than the control group.

Increase Longevity

Early studies on animals have found that an animal can experience an increased lifespan by including intermittent fasting. These studies found that even if animals had a higher body fat percentage than the control group, including intermittent fasting, they could increase their lifespan and longevity.

This makes sense, as intermittent fasting has many health benefits, and when all of these benefits are compounded together, it naturally results in a longer lifespan.

Lifestyle Ease

We all want to improve health and weight, but it is important also to have an easier lifestyle. When it is difficult to gain health and weight, many of us fail, as life is already busy and difficult enough without adding added worry and tasks. If a person cooks more, eats more frequently, and always worries about a diet, they are unlikely to stick to it, as it is merely unmaintainable.

It supports the secretion of the growth hormone

It's present in kids more than in grown-ups, but it still helps a lot. The growth hormone decreases fat and improves the development of bone and muscles. It does this by turning glycogen into glucose in the bloodstream. This enables fat burn without the reduction of muscles. When you sleep and exercise enough, the growth hormone is also boosted.

It enables you to avoid heart illnesses

Both blood glucose control and fat loss are done by IF to improve heart health. The likelihood of getting coronary artery heart illness can also be reduced.

Intermittent fasting is very versatile and can fit in any schedule

It is not as challenging as certain diets that unnecessarily trigger a huge disturbance in your life. There is no particular time to perform the IF. They can be blended as you think it is appropriate for your timetable. You are not boxed into any regiment that you cannot retain easily. Intermittent rapidity adapts to life's unpredictability. This can also be practiced everywhere globally as there is no special gear you need to do; it only restricts your feeding and is therefore much easier and more practical than many diets. It's completely all right, even if you have to halt fasting for a while. In a matter of minutes, you can begin fasting again.

It accepts all food

Organic foods have more nutrients than processed foods. These organic products are unfortunately quite costly, so purchasing them will diminish your pockets every day. They can be almost 10 times more expensive than processed products. It is easier to afford processed products as they are cheap. No matter the effectiveness of a diet, it cannot help you if you can't afford it. Fasting is in the first position of cost-effectiveness since it is completely free. You don't have to purchase any meals, so it costs you no cash. There's no reason you purchase costly meals or supplements or any drug that makes it cheap for all.

Simple to practice

Intermediate fasting is easy to do and doesn't have any complicated scheduling, it is quite direct. This causes it to be simpler to pursue and more efficient than many diets.

Opens up your mind

It enables you to regulate your mental procedures as IF opens up your body. You are used to responding to your body's urges because you consume whenever you feel slightly hungry. You are released from the control of your body as a result of practicing IF.

Corrects insulin resistance

This is the simplest and easiest route to reduce insulin resistance and insulin levels. It has a highly effective impact. It works better than a rigid low-carb diet.

Improves your metabolism

Intermittent fasting enhances your metabolism by considerably reducing the number of calories you eat in one day. During the feeding time you have, it is almost possible to eat the suggested daily calorific requirements. This causes modifications in the body and fat burning. It also helps you burn fat, even if you eat the normal calories your system requires, as it will make you burn fat for power instead of carbs.

Chapter 3: IF and Hormones

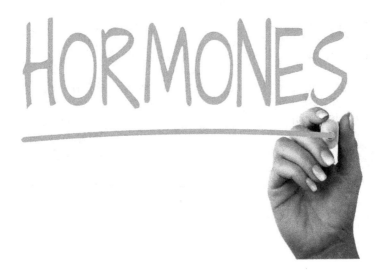

Upon reaching the age of 30, the aging process starts, and the body's hormones fluctuate. The process is different for everyone depending on genetics and several environmental factors, as men and women have different phases in their lives that affect the levels of their hormones. The human growth hormone is produced by the pituitary gland and contributes to adolescents' growth and development. The deficiency of human growth hormone in an adult means higher body fat and reduced muscle mass and bone density. Once it is availed from the pituitary gland, the human growth hormone only lasts a short time in the blood. From there, it finds its way to the liver where it is metabolized and initiated into growth factors.

That would be the same, which is linked to high insulin levels that lead to several health issues. However, the brief instance of the growth factors from human growth hormone lasts only a few minutes. All of the hormones are secreted naturally and done so in brief bursts to prevent the initiation of some resistance, which happens when the body gets used to high levels of the hormone in the bloodstream without acting proportionately to their secretion. The first discoveries of human growth hormone came from experiments on cadavers done in the 50s though it was synthesized in a lab environment during the 80s. After that, it became very popular as a performance-enhancing supplement. The normal levels of the hormone in a person tend to reach a peak during puberty as expected, and they gradually decrease afterward. Growth hormone tends to be produced when a person is sleeping and is one of the counter-regulatory hormones produced naturally. Both cortisol and HGH increase the level of glucose in the bloodstream by breaking down the glycogen to counters the effects that are rendered by insulin. Insulin reduces the amount of blood glucose levels while HGH increases blood glucose.

These hormones are usually secreted in pulses before a person wakes up. This would be deemed normal and it is supposed to get the body ready for the day by pushing the glucose out of storage and into the bloodstream where it is then available for energy creation. When someone says that a person needs to eat their breakfast to have the right energy levels for the day, this is very incorrect. The body has already provided enough resources for this to happen so there is no need to do cereals or a heavy breakfast to get the fuel needed for the day. This is why hunger happens to be its lowest during the early morning even if someone has not eaten during the night unless the body has already been conditioned to consume food during this time, which happens with most people.

Fasting to Increase the Levels of the Growth Hormone

In 1982, Kerndt produced a study that was of a single patient and they went through a 40-day fast for religious needs. The glucose levels decreased, from a level of 96, it dropped to a level of 56. The insulin went much lower and stabilized. The concern was the HGH though. According to the study, it started at a level of 0.74 and peaked at 9.86. That would mean a 1,250% increase in the level of the growth hormone. Even a fast for five days gives a significant increase in the growth hormone.

This is all according to research done on the subject. The question then goes to the potential side effects of the increased growth hormone from fasting. There might be an increased level of blood sugar for someone but there is hardly a risk for the potential of debilitating lifestyle diseases such as cancer and diabetes.

Fasting is seen as one of the great stimulating factors for HGH secretion. During the time of fasting, there happens to be a spike during the morning period, but there is usually some secretion going on during the day. The HGH is crucial after all to maintain and develop muscle fiber and bone density. Though, some of the main issues that come with fasting include the decreased levels of muscle mass. Some say fasting a single day would even cause a loss of about ¼ of a pound of muscle. The opposite is said to happen according to verified research. In comparing the caloric reduction diets to fasting, the fasting was much better at preserving lean mass.

Say that somebody is living during the prehistoric Paleolithic era. During the summer when food is abundant, the community would engage in a lot of feasting and then store some of that as fat within the body. During the time of winter, there would be nothing to eat. The question is whether the body would metabolize the muscle but preserve the stored fat. In this case, the body would burn the stored fat instead of the precious muscle fiber. It is true though that some protein is catabolized for gluconeogenesis purposes, though the increase in HGH maintains lean mass during the time of fasting.

The increases in human growth hormone when a person is fasting assist in preserving the muscle tissue and glycogen stores while using the fat stores instead. This breakdown of the fat in a process known as lipolysis releases glycerol and other fatty acids, which would be metabolized to create energy. Madelon Buijs, a researcher at the Leiden University Medical Center in the Netherlands, claims the increases in HGH rise noticeably during the first 13 hours of beginning a fast, which would mean an increased breakdown of fats in the first half of the day of the fast.

Blood Levels of Human Growth Hormone

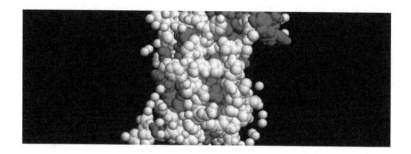

When fasting, loss of protein from the muscles increases by 50 percent in the cases of a lack of human growth hormone. Though, fasting and exercise during the fast may increase the levels of growth hormone. They are also subject to a lot of variation during the day because the pituitary gland releases the hormone in particular bursts. The random evaluation of the levels of human growth hormone as opposed to monitoring it overtime is not necessarily useful. Though, levels during the morning would be much higher than those recorded during the day.

36

Implications for the Athletes

This has significant ramifications for the athletes as it is known as training during the fasting phase. The increase of adrenaline from fasting will increase motivation so that the person will train harder. Similarly, the increased HGH levels as stimulated by the intermittent fasting will result in a toning effect and an increase in muscle mass that will help make recovery from the workout sessions that much easier. That would be a significant advantage for the athletes, especially in the endurance department. There is also a lot of new attention given to this approach to muscle treatment and exercise. It is not luck that many of the early proponents in training during the fasting state are bodybuilders. This is because it is a sport that requires a lot of high-intensity training and very low levels of body fat.

Even a book was written by bodybuilder Brad Pilon known as 'Eat, Stop, Eat'—which popularized the lean gains approach to fasting. For those individuals who believed fasting would increase fatigue levels and make you tired or it would not be possible to exercise during fasting, that is a wrong mentality. Fasting in itself does not cause you to burn muscle fiber significantly. There is no typical approach, meaning you have to shrivel up into a skeleton to get effective results from the fasted state. The difference with those scenarios is the individuals illustrated did not receive any form of nourishment during their fasts. They could even go weeks without sufficient water and food between days. At that level, you would be punishing your body rather than taming it and the situations are due to lack rather than an active choice because no one can hold out that long.

As such, fasting when done right has good potential in creating anti-aging properties brought about by human growth hormone without the potential problems created by excess HGH such as increased blood pressure and prostate cancer. For those interested in competing at an elite or athletic level, then the benefits would be much better for them.

Additional Information

The testing that comes with HGH is not particularly routine. At times, it is done to help diagnose the pituitary issues that can sometimes lead to conditions like gigantism or stunted growth. Even though HGH therapy is approved when it comes to treating those children that have stunted growth, it has also attracted a lot of attention because of the effects that it has been deemed to have on muscle and fat tissues. Synthetic HGH is available for purchase though not a lot is known about the long-term safety it has on the subject.

Chapter 4: Myths to Disprove About Intermittent Fasting

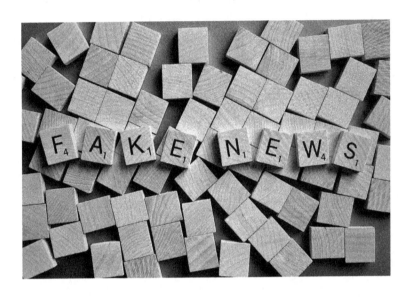

Issues that are not popular can be misunderstood with a lot of misconceptions and myths surrounding them. Intermittent fasting is one such issue. Many people with half-baked information suddenly become experts on the topic and are always willing to advise anyone willing to listen. It doesn't matter how long a false premise is considered correct, once the evidence is present, the error is exposed, and wise people will know to stick with the facts.

Myth 1: Intermittent Fasting is Unsafe for Older Adults

Anyone can engage in intermittent fasting as long as they do not have any medical conditions and are not pregnant or lactating. Of course, our bodies do not all have the same tolerance levels even in people that look exactly alike. If one or more persons respond negatively to intermittent fasting because they are advanced in age and are women, it does not mean that another will react the same way.

There is no doubt that intermittent fasting is not meant for everyone. Fasting is not safe for children because they need all the food they can get for continual development. Fasting in itself is not an issue for older people – any adult can fast.

Myth 2: You Gain Weight as You Age

A myth is a combination of facts and falsehood. This is a typical example of that. It is saying that growing older means your metabolism will slow down and your body will not burn or use up calories as fast as when you were younger. However, weight gain in older adults is not a given. The key to keeping your body performing optimally is to develop and maintain healthy habits such as fasting intermittently, drinking enough water, reducing stress levels, and getting adequate exercise.

Myth 3: Your Metabolism Slows Down During Fasting

This myth represents one of those big misunderstandings I mentioned earlier. The difference between calorie restriction and deliberately choosing when to take in calories is huge. Intermittent fasting does not necessarily limit calorie intake neither does it make you starve. It is when a person starves or under-eats that changes occur in their metabolic rate. But there is no change whatsoever in your metabolism when you delay eating for a few hours by fasting intermittently.

Myth 4: You Will Get Fat if You Skip Breakfast

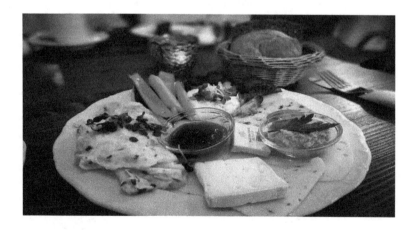

"Breakfast is the most important meal of the day!" This is one of the more popular urban myths about intermittent fasting. It is in the same category with the myths, "Santa doesn't give you presents if your naughty," and "carrots give you night vision." Some people will readily point to a relative or friend who is fat because they don't eat breakfast. But the question is: are they fat because they don't eat breakfast? Or do they skip breakfast because they are fat and want to reduce their calorie intake?

The best way to collect unbiased data when conducting scientific studies is through randomized controlled trials (RTC). After a careful study of 13 different RTCs on the relationship weight gain and eating or skipping breakfast, researchers from Melbourne, Australia found that both overweight and normal-weight participants who ate breakfast gained more weight than participants who skipped breakfast. The researchers also found that there's a higher rate of calorie consumption later in the day in participants who ate breakfast. This puts a hole in the popular notion that skipping breakfast will make people overeat later in the day (Harvard Medical School, 2019).

The truth is, there is nothing spectacular about eating breakfast as far as weight management is concerned. There is limited scientific evidence disproving or supporting the idea that breakfast influences weight. Instead, studies only show that there is no difference in weight loss or gain when one eats or skips breakfast.

Myth 5: Exercise Is Harmful to Older Adults Especially While Fasting

No. It is not harmful to exercise while fasting. And no, exercise is not harmful to older adults, whether they are fasting or not. On the contrary, exercising during your fasting window helps to burn stored fats in the body. When you perform physical activities after eating, your body tries to burn off new calories that are ingested from your meal. But when you exercise on an empty or nearly empty stomach, your body burns fats that are stored already and keeps you fit.

What is harmful to older adults is not engaging in exercises at all. A lack of exercise or adequate physical activity in older adults is linked to diabetes, heart disease, and obesity among other health conditions.

Researchers from Harvard Medical School demonstrated in a landmark study that frail and older women could regain functional loss through resistance exercise (Harvard Medical School, 2007). For ten weeks, participants from a nursing home (100 women aged between 72 and 98) performed resistance exercises three times a week. At the end of 10 weeks, the participants could walk faster, further, climb more stairs, and lift a great deal of weight than their inactive counterparts. Also, a 10-year study of healthy aging by researchers with the MacArthur Study of Aging in America found that older adults (people between 70 and 80 years) can get physically fit whether or not they have been exercising at their younger age. The bottom line is, as long as you can move the muscles in your body, do it because it is safe and will only help you live a better and longer life.

Myth 6: Eating Frequently Reduces Hunger

There is mixed scientific evidence in this regard. Some studies show that eating frequently reduces hunger in some people. On the other hand, other studies show the exact opposite. Interestingly, at least one study shows no difference in the frequency of eating and how it influences hunger (US National Library of Medicine, 2013). Eating can help some people get over cravings and excessive hunger, but there is no shred of evidence to prove that it applies to everyone.

Myth 7: You Can't Teach an Old Dog New Tricks

The brain never stops learning neither does it stop developing at any age. New neural pathways are created when a person learns something new at any age. And with continued repetition, the neural pathways become stronger until the behavior is habitual. Older people are often more persistent and have a higher motivation than younger people when it comes to learning new things. Learning should be a lifelong pursuit and not an activity reserved for young people.

Don't allow anyone to convince you into believing that it is too late to learn new eating habits because you are in your golden years or are approaching it. It doesn't matter if you've never tried fasting you can still train your brain to make fasting a habit even in old age. Start small, make it a natural occurrence in everyday life, repeating until you get used to it, and your positive results aka glowing skin, improved energy will motivate you to make it into a lifestyle.

Myth 8: You Must Lose Weight during Intermittent Fasting

This myth is rooted in the hype that intermittent fasting has received in recent years. Unless done correctly, intermittent fasting may not yield weight loss benefits. For you to experience any significant loss in weight, you must ensure that you eat healthily during your eating window. Equally, it is important to stick to the fasting schedule. If you keep cheating and adjusting your fasting window to favor more eating time or you overeat during the eating window to compensate for lost meals, your chances of losing weight will be greatly diminished.

Myth 9: Your Body Will Go Into "Starvation Mode" If You Practice Intermittent Fasting

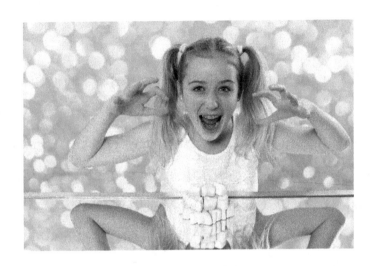

This myth is based on the misconception of what the starvation mode is and what triggers it. First of all, starvation is when your body senses that there is a significant drop in energy supply and reduces your metabolic rate. In simple terms, it is a reduction in the rate at which your body burns fat as a lack of food. This is an automatic response to conserve energy. It makes sense to reduce energy consumption if there is little to no supply of further energy coming from meals. In other words, if you stay away from food for too long, your body activates the starvation mode and significantly stops any further loss of body fat.

Having said that, intermittent fasting does not trigger the starvation mode. Instead, intermittent fasting helps to increase your metabolic activities. Meaning, your body can burn more fat when you fast for short periods. Starvation mode is only triggered when you engage in prolonged fasting over 48 hours, a practice I do not recommend for older adults.

Myth 10: An Aging Skin is Better Taken Care of with Anti-Aging Cream

This is not necessarily true. Brown spots, sagging skin, and wrinkles can indeed be reversed using expensive creams and topical treatments especially if a dermatologist prescribes them. These topical products exfoliate the top layer of your skin and make them appear smoother. However, that result (clear, smooth skin) is only a temporary effect.

A better way to look younger without any side effects is by activating autophagy. Engaging in mild stress-inducing activities such as intermittent fasting and exercising are the way. One key element to maintaining healthy skin is quenching your skin's thirst. Not drinking enough water can damage skin causing it to become dry, blemished, and lead to wrinkles. Drinking adequate amounts of water every day is the best approach to successfully "take the years off."

Myth 11: Fasting Deprives Your Brain of Adequate Dietary Glucose

Some people believe that your brain will underperform if you don't eat foods rich in carbohydrates. This myth is rooted in the notion that your brain uses only glucose as its fuel. But your brain doesn't use only dietary glucose for fuel. Some very low-carb diets can cause your body to produce ketone bodies from high-fat foods. Your brain can function well on ketone bodies. Continuous, intermittent fasting coupled with exercise can trigger the production of ketone bodies. Additionally, your body can also use a process known as gluconeogenesis to produce the sugar needed by your brain. This means that your body can effectively produce it on its own without you feeding it with just carbs.

Intermittent fasting does not interfere with brain function or its fuel or energy needs. However, because intermittent fasting is not suitable for everyone, if you feel shaky, dizzy, or extremely fatigued during fasting, consider talking with your doctor or reducing your fasting window.

Myth 12: Intermittent Fasting Will Make Older Adults Lose Their Muscle

First of all, it is stereotypical and largely incorrect to think of older people as frail. Frailty is not limited to just older adults and is a generalization of old age. Younger people can become frail if they suffer from a disabling chronic disease or have a poor diet. Scientists studied data from almost half a million people and found that middle-aged adults as young as 37 show signs of frailty (Mail Online, 2018).

Chapter 5: What to Eat and Not to Eat During Intermittent Fasting

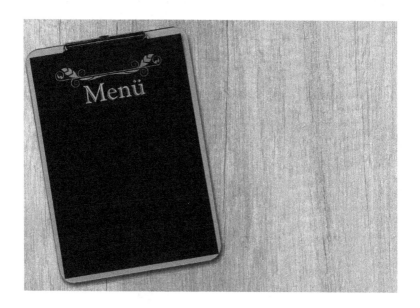

No matter how you plot your path when it comes to an intermittent fast, you need to have an understanding of what is good to eat, and not to eat during your efforts. Unless you are engaging in a complete fast from solid foods for 24 hours, you will have to know just what you should eat on your fast days. Likewise, it would be good to know what might be best suited for your non-fast days too. Because remember, just because you might be on one of your non-fast days, doesn't mean it would be a good idea to go downtown and binge at all you can eat buffet. Here in this chapter, we will help guide you to make wise food choices on what to eat and what not to eat during your intermittent fasting.

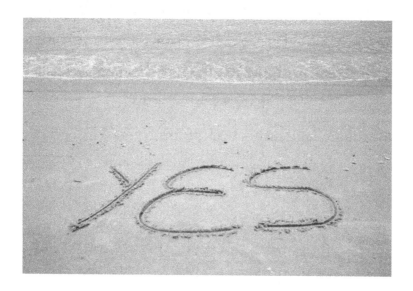

Coffee

Okay, well it's not really a food, but coffee as a zero-calorie beverage is a great supplement to any fast day. Most of us can't do without a cup of coffee in the morning as it is, so this is most certainly good news for those of us who enjoy our cup of morning joe. Coffee can also help to ameliorate possible negative reactions to fasting. If your initial fast has you feeling a bit lethargic and lacking in energy, for example, a good stiff cup of coffee could certainly help to offset those symptoms. But keep in mind that the coffee needs to be taken straight out of the pot, foregoing any creams or sugars. For some of you, unsweetened coffee just might have to be an acquired taste, but if you ditch the sugars and creams, you will be a lot better off in the long run.

Raspberries

Raspberries are a low-calorie food that won't wreck your fast day and at the same time, will help keep you regular by giving you a healthy dose of fiber. Raspberries also come replete with healthy vitamins and minerals, as well as inflammation-busting antioxidants. This is good to ward off arthritis and other degenerative conditions. In some situations, raspberries are even said to prevent cancer. This is due to the powerful cancer-busting phytochemicals it boasts, called "ellagic acid." At any rate, if you have nothing else to eat on a fast day, a bowl of plain, simple, raspberries would be a good dietary choice to make.

Low-Calorie Beans and Legumes

Beans, beans, the magical fruit. The more you eat, the more fat you can burn for your fast. Both beans and legumes are packed with healthy nutrients and are typically low in calories. They also have plenty of protein, helping to keep your muscles fueled even while your fat stores are depleted. Tiny but mighty, beans and legumes are fully capable of aiding in the process of weight reduction, during your intermittent fast. Most especially good when it comes to intermittent fasting are peas, black beans, lentils, and garbanzo beans.

Blueberries

These fruitful treats are low in calories yet high in antioxidants, helping to ensure the body remains free of nasty free radicals that could degrade bodily tissue over time. Blueberries are known immune boosters too, good for ensuring you don't get sick or otherwise compromised while you fast. Another neat thing about blueberries is that they contain a little something called flavonoids, which if consumed over a long period of time, can work to reduce overall BMI (Body Mass Index). This is most definitely a good thing. And did I mention? They also taste great!

Eggs

Whether you hard boil them, scramble them, or poach them—the incredible, edible egg is a great low calorie, nutrient-dense food for your fast days. Eggs just seem especially geared for this task. Eggs have a ton of proteins and tend to stick with you, leaving you feeling full and satisfied. If you are indeed allowing a small allotment of under 500 calories on your fast day, adding a couple of eggs to the mix certainly won't ruin your fast.

Lean Chicken Breast

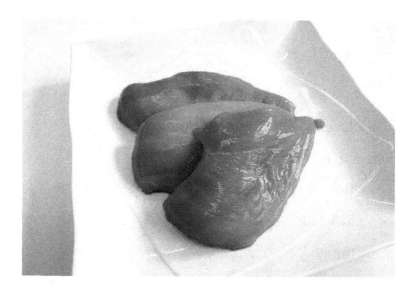

If you aren't doing a 24 hour fast, a serving of lean chicken breast is a good way to end a fast day that shouldn't exceed your 500-calorie allotment. Lean chicken breast provides plenty of proteins without all the filler of other sides of the meat. It's also a mainstay that goes well with quite a few meals and recipes. Here, in this book for one, you will find plenty of dishes that make full use of the power of a piece of lean chicken. Having that said, you should definitely stock up on some lean chicken breast in preparation for your next intermittent fast.

Fish

Just like chicken, fish is a good source of protein and yet won't break your budget of allotted calories on your fast day. Fish has a ton of what are known as omega-3 fatty acids. Don't let the "fat" word scare you though because omega-3 fatty acids are a good thing. There's a reason why every health food store has aisle after aisle of omega-3 supplements. Because its omega-3 fatty acids can safeguard our heart, dramatically reduce blood pressure, clear out plaque from arteries, and even prevent heart attacks and strokes. Fish is also considered a "brain food" due to its ability to help enhance cognitive function. Fish—it's decidedly nutritious, and it's downright delicious! Be sure to make use of it.

Veggies

You don't have to be a vegetarian to appreciate the tremendous benefit that veggies can provide. Vegetables represent a stabilizing force on your non-fast day and every day between. As well as providing plenty of valuable nutrients, veggies also give us a healthy dose of fiber to help keep us regular. Vegetables are typically low in calories too, so you can mix and match them with all kinds of meals regardless of meal plans. Be sure to have plenty of fresh veggies on hand.

Whole Grains

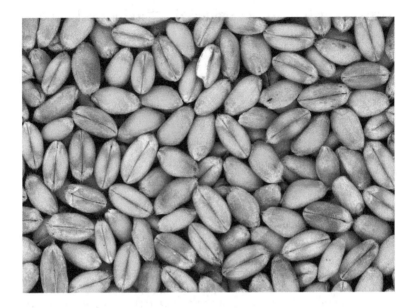

Whole grains are a great source of nutrition on fast or non-fast day either one. Unlike refined grains that spike your insulin, these morsels won't make you mess up your fast, and will still leave you feeling full and satisfied. You will find quite a few recipes in this book that make use of whole grain. It makes for a good bread alternative, so if you are ever in doubt— just reach for the whole grains!

Yogurt

When people think of healthy foods, one of the first things that come to mind is probably yogurt. Yogurt is an excellent source of nutrients and also provides a boost to your metabolism and energy even as you fast. Yogurts also come complete with a dose of probiotics that once ingested will work around the clock to keep your gut in good shape. The experts are stressing more and more that so-called good gut bacteria is the key to good health. Having that said, yogurt is a safe way to get plenty of it. Yogurt certainly does help when it comes to your preparation for your intermittent fasting regimen.

Dark Chocolate

I know not everyone is a fan of dark chocolate, and perhaps it's an acquired taste. But whether it takes you a while to appreciate it or not, the health benefits are immediate. Dark chocolate gives you a boost of energy even while fortifying your system with valuable antioxidants. The kind of antioxidants capable of fighting off cancer no less. Simply put, dark chocolate is some powerful stuff. With so much going for it, dark chocolate is a go-to food when it comes to intermittent fasting.

Coconut Oil

Coconut oil is a low-calorie, known metabolism booster, and will get your system up and running during your period of intermittent fasting. Coconut oil is good because it doesn't trigger insulin production unlike other oils do. You can use coconut oil as a supplement, or even a cooking aid, without any fear of disrupting your fast in the process. It's really quite a wonderful ingredient and you will see it made use of quite extensively in the recipes in this book.

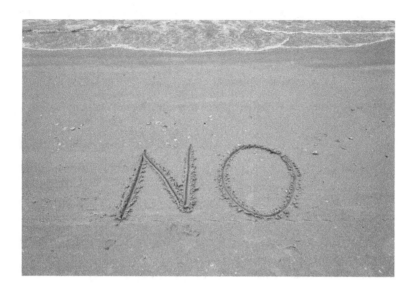

Soda

What no soda? You've got to be kidding me! Sorry folks, I like a good fountain drink of soda just like the next person, but I'm afraid it's all too true. If you want to engage in intermittent fasting, you are going to have to leave your soda behind. This is not meant as a punishment—it's simply the reality of the beast. One of the major components of an intermittent fast, after all, is the avoidance of sugar. It's so your body will start burning fat stores already in place that during fasting we refrain from guzzling sugary soda for our metabolic rate to nibble on. So yes, for the time being, as you engage in an intermittent fasting routine, you will indeed have to forego soda.

Heavily Processed Food

As you have probably already picked up during the course of this book, processed foods are frowned upon. Anything that has been processed and packaged is going to have a ton of preservatives packed into them, that while generally harmless, will have a long-term effect on your system over time. Heavily processed food will also pose a direct interference with your metabolism. That's why the fresher the food, the better when it comes to intermittent fasting.

Sugary Sweets

Just like with sugary sodas, sugary sweets would be completely counterproductive for an intermittent fast. The goal of an intermittent fast after all is to switch the body from burning sugar and carbs, to burning our latent fat deposits instead. Eating sugary sweets would disrupt this process and instead just add more junk to the fat already deposited in our trunk. So yes, you must avoid sugary sweets at all costs while you participate in intermittent fasting.

Alcohol

I don't mean to be a party pooper or anything, but let me just go ahead and say it. Alcohol and intermittent fasting do not mix. The reason? Alcohol has a direct effect on fat-burning metabolism. And the last thing that you would want to do is wreck your fast by throwing a wrench in your fat-burning metabolism! Alcohol also carries, carbs, sugars, calories, and the like. So, yeah just like drinking and driving—drinking and fasting should be avoided.

Refined Grains

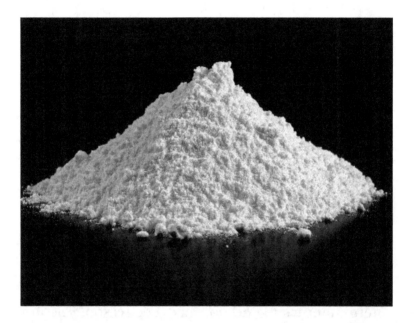

Unlike whole grains, refined grains will indeed have a decidedly negative impact on your fast. Refined grains once metabolized will actually turn directly into sugar. As already mentioned, a few times in this chapter, sugar will defeat the purpose of your fast.

The whole purpose of intermittent fasting is to get your body to stop burning sugar as fuel and burn fat instead. Ingesting refined grains that turn into sugar, therefore, completely negates this process. It will also raise your insulin levels. Having that said, refined grains are to be avoided if at all possible.

Trans-Fat

To be perfectly blunt, trans-fats are just bad. No good can come from them. And most especially, no good could come from your fast by ingesting them. Trans-fat, the fatty acids found in certain milk and meat products should be avoided while you participate in an intermittent fast. It raises, cholesterol, insulin, and wrecks any chance you may have had of having a successful fast. Just say no, when it comes to trans-fat.

Fast Food

Even though we call it "fast food"—the burgers and fries we bag from places like McDonald's are not exactly the best thing to eat during an intermittent fast! One look at an overly processed, carb-dense meal from McDonald's and I think you might probably understand why.

At any rate, presented here are the foods that you should and shouldn't eat. Take note and take heart. Enjoy your fast!

Chapter 6: The Right Mindset

We all know in the 21st century that wellbeing starts with healthy eating habits. Then why is it so difficult to stick to a balanced diet? The grocery store's aisles, posters on the doctor's offices, and even some TV advertisements use vivid colors and bold lettering to advertise healthy living. Women over 50 years are especially advised to watch what they eat as it is easier for them to gain weight than lose it.

The issue is not because people don't want to change their eating habits; it's that they don't even know how to do it. They get on board a new weight-loss plan, which they soon discard as such diets are often unsustainable when compared with regular lifestyles.

That's not the best way to go for a balanced lifestyle. Instead, you want to make a meaningful, permanent improvement, but you have to make sure you are doing it right. The guide below will help and show you how to stick to healthy eating habits. By setting realistic expectations and being persistent, you will find that good eating patterns are now well within your grasp even though they were impossible in the past. Each diet and weight-loss plan has its benefits and drawbacks, so you have to prepare your mind for it if you want to succeed.

The hardest factor in weight loss is changing your attitude about how to lose weight.

Many people attempt to lose weight with the worst imaginable mental state. They bolt into diets and workout programs out of personal-deprecation, all the while squeezing their "trouble" spots, branding themselves "fat" and feeling entirely less than that. They get distracted with results, rely on fast solutions, and lose sight of what good health is all about.

This kind of thought can be harmful. Instead of concentrating on the benefits that can come from weight loss—such as improved wellbeing, healthier life, greater satisfaction of daily lives, and the avoidance of diabetes and cardiac disease—these people focus on their pessimistic feelings. Eventually, poor thinking leads to disappointment.

Changing your mentality about weight loss goes beyond feeling-good; it's about the outcome. A study at the University of Syracuse indicates that the more unhappy women are with their bodies, the more likely they are to skip exercise. And just focusing on the fact that you're overweight is forecasting a potential weight gain—according to studies reported in the International Journal of Obesity in 2015.

Although psychologists emphasize that your actions are determined by how you view yourself and your core personality (seeing yourself as being overweight or undesirable makes you behave accordingly), genetics may also play a role. A study published in Psychosomatic Medicine journal also suggested that cortisol, the stress hormone, is secreted by the adrenal glands every time you get yourself down or think about your weight, which further causes weight gain.

It All Starts With Your Mindset

The problem with a lot of trendy diets is that they don't want you to think differently. They tell you to make a drastic adjustment to your eating habits. This is not healthy. If you are actively trying to change your eating habits, then first you have to fix your way of thinking about food.

Many people who are struggling to eat healthily have what researchers term a "closed mentality." These people believe that nothing can ever change, and they take this belief with them in beginning a new weight loss plan. They think that their health issues are simply the effects of poor biology, or that the embarrassment of solving the problem would reverse any improvements.

For certain people with a fixed mentality, long before it begins, a change of diet is futile. In reality, many would prefer to stay obese because it feels safer and less stressful than attempting to make a lifestyle change.

Unfortunately, anyone who wants to move to a healthier lifestyle without changing their attitude first will soon get discouraged. That's because the journey to a healthy lifestyle doesn't happen overnight. There are no magic foods, no matter what the magazine said or what some star did to shed baby weight or to dress for a new role. If you are someone with a fixed mindset starting a weight loss diet, you'll undoubtedly come to think the plan failed when you don't see any significant difference—reinforcing your original fears. The diet's failure will only make it harder for you to begin a new journey to eating healthy. There is another mindset that Psychologists refer to as a "growth mindset." While the fixed mindset believes little else can be changed, the growth mindset thinks things are continually evolving.

People with a growth mindset don't design their thoughts to be negative. Instead, they understand that small mistakes are just part of improvement. They realize that risks are only a minor problem in achieving something big. Therefore, people with a growth mindset recognize that progress needs incremental steps in the right direction, rather than resigning themselves to the inevitable.

What kind of attitude do you have? If you have a fixed mindset, how do you make the necessary change?

One of the easiest ways to begin making a change is by collecting information about the process. I highly recommend that you maintain a journal. This is so when you see subtle improvements leading up to a significant transition, they don't get lost. Start by writing down your expectations and record whether or not you have successfully met them.

A growth mindset is not a crazy dreamer mindset when it comes to goals. When setting your targets, always make sure that they are fair. Keep note of how many balanced meals you consume, relative to how many might not be. Act to increase the number of nutritious meals you consume each week.

You've got to understand more than anything that your mindset may be what held you off. The good news is that you're well on your way to make a meaningful difference when you know that mindset is part of the problem!

Below are some steps you can take to change your mindset.

Adjust your Priorities

The reason might be to lose weight, but that should not be the target. Instead, the objectives should be small, manageable stuff that you have full power to control. Have you consumed five fruit and veggie servings today? That's one goal achieved. What about 8 hours of sleep; have you got them in? If so, you can cross them off your list.

Gravitate to Positivity

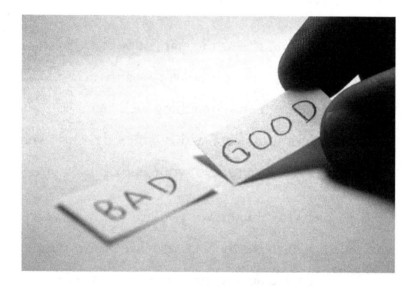

It is vital to Surround yourself with the Good. Doing so offers you a relaxing, socially healthy environment to invest in yourself. Don't be afraid to ask for help or support.

Rethink Punishments and Rewards

Remember that making healthier decisions is a way to practice self-care. Food is not a reward, and a workout is not a penalty. They are all necessary to take care of your body and to make you do the best you can. You deserve both.

Taking a few minutes at the start of your exercise or at the beginning of your day to calm down, and simply concentrate on breathing will help you set your goals, communicate with your body, and even reduce the stress response of your body.

Find a quiet space wherever you are (even at work), and try this exercise to help you feel more relaxed and ready to tackle the rest of your day. Lie with your legs outstretched on your back and put one hand on your stomach and one on your shoulder. Breathe in for four seconds through your nose, stay for two, and exhale for six seconds through your lips. Repeat this process for 5-10 minutes, focusing on the sensation of your stomach rising and falling with each breath.

24 Hour Goals

Having patience is essential when you are losing weight. Plus, if you concentrate on reaching genuinely reachable targets, such as taking 10.000 steps each day, you don't need to be caught up in your list of goals. New accomplishments come in every 24 hours; concentrate on those.

Like Bob Proctor says: "If you want to improve the quality of your life, start allocating a portion of each day to changing your paradigm."

Identify 'Troublesome Thoughts'

Identify the feelings that bring you problems, and seek to prevent and change them. Let them stop intentionally by saying 'no' out loud. It may sound silly, but that simple action breaks your chain of thought and helps you to introduce a new, safer one. The easiest way to do so is to count as many times as you like from one to 100 until your negative thoughts go away.

Don't step on the scale

Even though stepping on the scale to check on your progress is not bad, many people often associate it with negative thoughts. If you know the number on the scale will lead to negative and self-destructive thoughts, then you should avoid it. At least until you are in a place where the number on the scale doesn't affect your mental health.

Forget about the Entire 'Foods' attitude

We've learned somewhere along the way to feel either proud or bad for any food choice we make.

But in the end, it's just food, so you shouldn't feel bad for enjoying an occasional cookie. Permit yourself to have a piece of chocolate cake or a glass of wine sometimes.

Treating yourself to some comfort food is right for your mind and body. It is doing it every day that sabotages weight loss. During a more or less strict diet, having a day in a week to get away from is the key to success, the guarantee for motivation, and does not undermine the goal of losing weight.

Focus on the Attainable

If you've never been to a gym before, your goal on day one shouldn't be to do 30 minutes on the elliptical. Going for a 30-minute walk might be a better goal. If you want to cook more but have little familiarity with healthier cooking, don't bank on creating new nutritious recipes every night after work. Instead, consider using a subscription service such as Blue Apron or HelloFresh, where pre-portioned recipes and ingredients are delivered to your doorstep, helping you get to know different components, make new meals, and develop your cooking skills.

Envision a better life

What will life be like if you put good habits in place? Will you be more comfortable in your clothes? Will it give you more energy? Will you sleep better? Will you laugh more? Will you be happier? Will you be a better wife or mum? Attempt to get as thorough and realistic as possible. How will your life change if you changed your lifestyle?

Take a moment and sit down with a pen and ask yourself, what do I want? What do I really want? Write it down and make a written description of it in the present tense. Build a vision of what you would like to accomplish.

Take time to visualize a better life in the beginning and throughout your weight loss plan. Changing your habits is hard, so why bother if it doesn't bring you something new and better. Imagine a better life that will start giving you something to look forward to as well as work towards. See what you want, get a picture of it in your mind. Vision is going to direct your life.

Believe in your vision

This is important. There's no point in having a vision unless you think it will come true. With almost everything, you have to believe that you can make this happen. So you can change your lifestyle, lose weight, and hope for a better future. To be successful, you have to believe you can do it without anybody else's evaluation. You have to believe in what you see. Keep your vision up front, and think it's waiting for you. You have to persist and persevere in working on what you want to achieve. That'll keep you focused and move on.

Imagining a happier future makes you hopeful – although things go wrong sometimes, you will just have to hope it's for the greater good. Learning not to focus on the bad will help you stay focused on living a healthier lifestyle.

Sacrifice is giving up something of a lower nature, to receive something of a higher nature. Sacrifice is based on faith, and if you have faith, you will take action.

Believe you are in control

You must realize you control your life. You have to take responsibility for your actions to excel in losing weight and other goals – you have to trust that you are in charge. If you put your future in other people's hands, you will never be able to move on. Of course, there are always circumstances out of our control, but your type of reaction is up to you.

While taking control of your life is empowering, it's also frightening because if you don't achieve your goal, you have no one to blame but yourself. "No one has control over your life – but you."

Get to learn how to cope

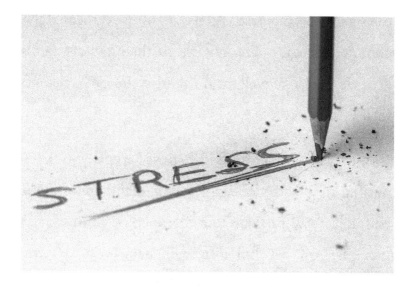

Many of your problems with weight loss are from your physiological reactions to stress. Most times, you crave spaghetti or candy when you have a bad day. Or you order a pizza because there was nothing to cook for dinner. Or give up on losing weight when work gets busy, or when you get to some other stressful season of life.

When you want to lose weight, life doesn't just continue effortlessly without stress. Sadly, life will never be secure, and there will always be a pain. Consequently, if you fall off track each time, life does not go your way, then it is time you learn new coping strategies. The goal is to maintain a healthy lifestyle and lose weight, no matter the obstacles life throws our way.

If the way you cope with stress keeps you from putting new behaviors in place or maintaining them, you might want to talk to a therapist or counselor. A therapist or psychologist will help you develop healthier coping skills and work through stress. This will help you free up space in your brain to focus on that better life. Having excellent optimistic coping

91

skills is necessary for growth and surviving – not just for weight loss. Life is unpredictable and will not always go according to plan. Either you can get better or get bitter.

"The secret of success is learning how to use pain and pleasure instead of having pain and pleasure use you. If you do that, you're in control of your life. If you don't, life controls you." Tony Robbins

Eliminate the clutter and the chaos

What do clutter and chaos have to do with weight loss? It's tough to picture a happier future when you are surrounded by confusion and noise. Clutter and confusion build hot zones, and when attempting to escape hot zones, it's challenging to develop new patterns and behaviors. Hot zones are moments when you feel stressed, overwhelmed, and the decisions you make are more about surviving the moment than on long-term goals.

Concentrate on solutions and not explanations

A proactive approach that has been effective in the weight loss process is relying on options instead of excuses. You may be using excuses because you're scared of failing. So you say something like, "I can't get to the gym at that time" or "I 'm sick" or "That exercise never worked for me" instead of falling into an exercise routine. It offers you the freedom to either give up or not try at all. Failure, however, is part of the process. Failure is Good. And instead of making yourself give up, grant yourself the approval to lose. To succeed, you have to be okay with failure, not just at losing weight but in life in general.

Chapter 7: Useful Supplements: Spirulina Algae

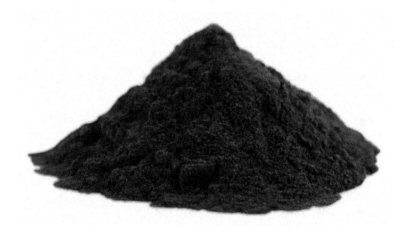

Spirulina (pronounced speer-uh-lee-nuh) is an edible type of cyanobacteria, a single-celled, blue-green microalgae that is found naturally in both salt and freshwaters. This spiral-shaped microalga is cultivated and harvested throughout the world as both a supplement and whole food. Because it has a soft cell wall made of protein and complex sugars, it can be digested efficiently. It is widely considered a green superfood with positive health benefits because of its richness in:

- Protein (dried spirulina contains between 50% to 70% protein)

- Minerals (especially Iron and Manganese)

- Vitamins (especially Vitamins B1, and B2)

- Carotenoids

- Antioxidants

Spirulina is used internationally in nutrition drinks, pasta, crackers, noodles, nutrition bars, broths, cakes, pet foods, and cereal. It is also used as a component in food coloring, cosmetics, skin creams, shampoos, personal care products, and more. Spirulina can be purchased at most specialty nutrition stores, some supermarket chains, as well as online. It is typically sold in powder or tablet form.

As a food, eating spirulina is nothing new. Historians indicate that spirulina was part of the diet of the Kanem Empire of Chad in the ninth century (AD/CE). In 1519, Hernando Cortez and his Spanish Conquistadors observed that spirulina was eaten by Aztecs around Lake Texcoco, which is modern-day Mexico City. Today, more than one thousand metric tons of spirulina are harvested worldwide in natural lakes, commercial farms, village farms, and family microfarms.

Spirulina farming is much more environmentally friendly compared to conventional food production. Most conventional foods are generated using chemicals including pesticides, antibiotics, preservatives, additives, and fungicides. Not only have these chemicals been shown to have negative impacts on health, but they also cause damage to our water supply and the overall natural environment. Harvesting spirulina offers more nutrition per acre, and doesn't incur environmental costs associated with toxic cleanup, water treatment, or subsidies, that other food industries require.

The growing popularity of spirulina as a green superfood has taken off over the past forty years. Scientific research conducted in recent decades support the many health benefits of spirulina, adding to its growing use as a food or supplement. Research is ongoing, and in some cases, has not been tested on human subjects. Additionally, the U.S. FDA has not approved spirulina as a medicine or treatment for diseases (although it is an approved supplement and food). However, the health benefits that research has uncovered so far have been very positive, showing some transformative results.

Cancer Fighter

Spirulina is high in beta-carotene, a type of phytochemical, that is believed to help protect the body against free radicals that can come from various forms of pollution including cigarette smoke and herbicides. The effects of spirulina on cancer have been demonstrated in animals and humans with positive effects indicating a reduction in cancer cells, and even in some cases, the reversal of oral cancer.

Diabetes and Blood Sugar Improvement

A study from the University of Baroda in India revealed that spirulina may help people with diabetes. Over the course of a two-month study, patients with type 2 diabetes who were given two grams of spirulina every day improved blood sugar and lipid levels.

Immune System Boost

Tests on animals and senior citizens have exhibited a boost of the immune system, which is crucial to preventing viral infections. In these studies, spirulina was shown to increase the production of antibodies, which are needed to fight viral and bacterial infections, as well as some chronic illnesses.

Anti-Virus

Not only has the algae been observed to boos antibodies, but it has also shown an ability to hinder the replication of viruses. The National Cancer Institute (NCI) publicized that spirulina was "remarkably active" against the AIDS virus (HIV-1) after conducting a study in 1989. Test tube experiments have also shown spirulina to inhibit the replication of other viruses including influenza A, mumps, and measles.

Antihistamine

In several scientific studies, spirulina appeared to help allergy symptoms such as watery eyes, skin reactions, and runny nose. In a recent study, a group of people suffering from rhinitis, an inflammation of

99

the nasal mucous membrane, saw significant improvements in their allergy symptoms when given a daily 1000mg or 2000mg doses of spirulina over the course of twelve weeks.

Blood Pressure Reduction

Participants in an experiment at the National Autonomous University of Mexico were able to drop their blood pressure after taking spirulina for six weeks, without any other changes in their diet. Spirulina increases the body's production of nitric oxide, which is a gas that can widen blood vessels. Widened blood vessels improve the body's flow of blood, and ultimately can reduce blood pressure.

Lower Cholesterol

Recent research conducted in Greek universities has shown some promising effects on adults with high cholesterol. Over the course of three months, fifty-two adults were given one gram of spirulina each day. At the end of the three-month study period, the group's average triglycerides decreased over 16% and low-density lipoprotein (LDL) cholesterol (also known as the "bad" cholesterol) by 10%.

Radiation Treatment

After the Russian Chernobyl nuclear disaster in 1986, the Russian government turned to spirulina to treat children who had been exposed to radiation. Radiation destroys bone marrow, thus complicating the body's ability to create normal white or red blood cells. Within six weeks, children who were fed five grams of spirulina every day were able to make remarkable recoveries. The blue pigment of spirulina is comprised of phycocyanin, which enables the body to cleanse some radioactive metals.

Kidney and Liver Detoxification

Not only has spirulina's phycocyanin been shown to cleanse radioactive metals, but it may also have the ability to cleanse heavy metal poisoning. Studies in Japan and elsewhere suggest that spirulina is able to safely assist in the removal of heavy metals such as arsenic, lead, mercury, and other similar metals that can be found in medicine, dental fillings, fish, deodorants, cigarettes, and drinking water.

Reducing Malnutrition

According to the United Nations Food and Agricultural Organization, over 800 million people worldwide suffer from chronic undernourishment. Malnutrition is an epidemic as millions of people around the world lack enough proteins and micronutrients such as vitamins and minerals. With spirulina containing a significant amount of protein, B-vitamins, and iron, one tablespoon a day could eliminate micronutrient deficiencies that cause diseases such as anemia. Unlike other protein foods such as beef or nuts, spirulina is a very digestible source of protein. The digestive tract of malnourished individuals exhibits malabsorption, making the easily digestible spirulina, an even more attractive source of nourishment.

Conclusion

As you can see, there are numerous benefits that come with employing an intermittent fasting diet. After reading this book, you now have this information and much, much more! You are fully equipped to begin changing your life with programs designed specifically for you, and I hope that you feel empowered to do so!

The main takeaway from this book is that there are many options for women over the age of 50 to take control of their weight loss strategies without having to turn to methods designed for men or people in their twenties. Further, taking control of your health and playing an active role in your disease risk reduction is not as difficult as it sounds. I hope that after reading this book, you have a new understanding of what you can do and how your body will react, given your age and sex.

As you take all of this information forth with you, it may seem overwhelming to begin applying this to your own life. Remember, life is a process, and you do not need to expect perfection from yourself. By reading this book, you are already on your way to changing your life. If you fall off of the diet and you need inspiration, come back to the first chapters of this book and remind yourself why you wanted to begin it in the first place.

Many thanks for completing this book. I hope it was practical enough and able to provide you with the vital tools you need to attain your fitness goals.

CPSIA information can be obtained
at www.ICGtesting.com
Printed in the USA
LVHW082224210321
682037LV00002B/48